Getting Over the Love Affair with Food

How Important is Living to You?

Amir Carter

Mid Atlanta Book Publishing

Getting Over the Love Affair with Food: How Important Is Living to You?

ISBN: 979-8-9936892-1-0

Published by **Mid Atlanta Book Publishing** Atlanta, Georgia.

Contents

Dedication

This book is dedicated to my parents, Calvin and Nelda. Two of the most important and influential people in my life. Your love, strength, and wisdom have shaped the person I am today.

You taught me self-confidence, self-love, respect, and compassion for others. Through your example and incredible sacrifices, you showed me what it means to live with purpose and to give back.

Because of you, I am able to help others on their journey of healing and growth.

Forever grateful.

Introduction

Why does this book matter? Because life itself depends on how we treat our bodies. The modern world has turned food into a trap: fast food, chemicals, preservatives, and addictive flavors. The result? A society full of obesity, diabetes, heart disease, and stress.

But there is another path. A path of healing through fasting, clean eating, herbs, exercise, and respect for the body. This book will guide you step by step on how to break the chains of unhealthy habits and return to balance.

In today's world, food is everywhere. It is advertised on billboards, flashing across television screens, pushed into our phones, and stocked on every corner. The majority of this food, however, is not designed to nourish your body. It is designed to get you hooked. Companies invest billions into engineering flavors that hijack your brain, textures that make you crave more, and packaging that makes you believe what you're buying is "healthy" when in truth, it is filled with chemicals and preservatives.

The result? A society drowning in poor health. Diabetes, obesity, heart disease, cancer, and digestive illnesses have become normal. People live with constant fatigue, mood swings, and inflammation, often without realizing that much of it begins with what they are putting in their mouths.

Writing Breaking the Love Affair with Food has been one of the most personal and eye-opening experiences of my life. This book was born out of my own journey of learning, healing, and understanding the powerful relationship we all have with food. For many of us, food has become more than nourishment. It has become comfort, company, or even a way to cope with life's pain and pressure.

For years, I believed that controlling what I ate was the answer. But I eventually realized it wasn't about control. It was about connections. Real healing began when I started asking deeper questions: Why do I crave certain foods? What am I trying to fill? What emotions am I avoiding? And most importantly, how much of my life am I missing by being disconnected from my true self?

This book isn't about guilt or perfection. It's about awareness, compassion, and the courage to face what's underneath our choices. I want readers to know that they are not alone. Every step forward, no matter how small, is a victory.

Through these pages, I hope to inspire you to look within, to rebuild your relationship with food, and to rediscover your love for life. Because when we learn to truly nourish ourselves physically, mentally, and spiritually, we begin to experience freedom in its truest form. If you have ever asked yourself, "How important is living to me?" This book will help you answer this question with action.

Chapter One

Breaking the Love Affair with Food

Most people do not realize it, but food is not just a source of nourishment. It has become an emotional relationship. For some, food is a comforter after a stressful day. For others, it is a reward, a distraction, or even a form of self-punishment. This emotional attachment creates what I call a "love affair with food." And like many toxic relationships, it can keep you trapped in cycles of pleasure and pain.

Think about it: how many times have you eaten when you weren't hungry, simply because you were bored, sad, or celebrating? How often have you reached for sweets or snacks to soothe your emotions? This pattern is not entirely your fault. Food companies deliberately design processed foods to be addictive. Sugar, artificial flavorings, and chemical enhancers light up the brain's reward centers, much like drugs do. The more you eat, the more your brain demands.

Breaking this love affair begins with awareness. You must learn to pause and ask yourself: Am I eating because I am hungry, or because I am seeking comfort? True hunger is steady and patient. It does not scream or demand junk food. Emotional hunger, on the other hand, is sudden, urgent, and specific. You don't just "want food," you want chips, cookies, ice cream or soda. That is not hunger; that is a craving rooted in habit and addiction.

The solution is not to starve yourself or live in restriction. The solution is mindfulness. Slow down and pay attention to what you are eating and how it makes you feel. Chew your food thoroughly. Notice the texture, the flavors, the effect it has on your body. Stop eating when you are satisfied, not when you are stuffed. Food should be a tool for nourishment, not an emotional crutch. Ending the love affair with food is the first step toward freedom. It requires honesty and discipline, but once you break those chains, you will discover something powerful: food tastes better when it is no longer controlling you.

Food is life, but for many of us it has become a relationship. Like a romance that begins with sweetness and comfort, our love affair with food often ends in heartbreak: disease, fatigue, and regret. This chapter is about waking up to that relationship and learning how to let go of the toxic bond we've created with what we eat.

Food Is More Than Hunger

We live in a world where eating is rarely just about survival. Food is tied to:

- Emotions – We eat when we're stressed, sad, or celebrating.
- Culture – Every holiday, gathering, or tradition is built around meals.
- Comfort – We turn to certain foods for nostalgia and safety.

None of these are wrong on their own, but when food becomes the primary way we deal with life, we fall into dependence. That's when food stops being medicine and becomes poison. Food companies know this. They spend billions on designing foods that hijack our brain chemistry. Sugar, fat, and salt are carefully engineered to trigger dopamine, the same "pleasure" chemical released when people gamble, drink, or take drugs. Here's why. The food is designed to own you.

- Potato chips are "addictive."

- Fast food always tastes the same.
- Candy bars leave you wanting another one.

The Cycle of Control

When we're in love with food, the cycle looks like this:

- Craving hits.
- We eat to satisfy emotions, not hunger.
- Temporary comfort comes, but guilt follows.
- The body weakens from processed chemicals.
- The cycle repeats.

This isn't living. It's bondage!

***

Learning Mindful Eating

Breaking the love affair with food doesn't mean never enjoying a meal again. It means taking back control. Try this practice:

- Pause before eating. Ask: "Am I hungry or just triggered?"
- Eat slowly. Put the fork down between bites.
- Listen to your body. Notice how food makes you feel. Not just while eating, but hours later.
- Stop at satisfied, not stuffed. Fullness is your body's way of saying, that's enough.

Food is meant to support life, not dominate it.

***

Redefining the Relationship

Like leaving a toxic romance, ending the love affair with food requires boundaries. It means:

- Setting limits (no eating after 9 PM).
- Choosing better partners (fresh, whole foods instead of processed ones).
- Finding new sources of joy (exercise, meditation, healthy food, juicing, creativity, positive connections).

You deserve to live free, not chained to cravings.

***

Action Steps for Chapter 1

1. Write down the top three foods you crave most. Be honest.
2. Track when you crave them. Late at night? After stress? While bored?
3. Replace one of those foods with a healthier option this week.
4. Practice mindful eating at one meal a day.

Chapter Two

Timing Matters - When to Stop Eating

One of the most powerful healing tools available to us costs nothing at all: fasting. For thousands of years, fasting has been practiced for both spiritual and physical renewal. Ancient cultures understood that giving the body periods of rest allowed it to repair itself. Modern science is finally catching up, confirming what our ancestors knew: fasting heals.

When you stop eating at 9:00 PM, something amazing happens. Instead of spending energy digesting food, your body switches into repair mode. Hormones that help burn fat and restore cells begin to activate. In the morning, by skipping breakfast and delaying your first meal until 12 PM (or 11 AM for those who need to take medication), you extend this repair window even further. This is called intermittent fasting, and it is one of the simplest, most effective ways to restore balance to the body.

During fasting hours, insulin levels drop. Lower insulin allows your body to tap into stored fat for energy. At the same time, processes like autophagy, your body's natural detox system, kick in. Autophagy literally means "self-eating," and while it may sound strange, it is the process by which your body breaks down damaged cells and recycles them. This is the very essence of anti-aging and disease prevention.

But fasting is not just about weight loss or vanity. It is about giving your digestive system a chance to rest. In our modern world, people eat around the clock. Snacking in the car, at the desk, late at night in front of the television. The gut is constantly overloaded, and when it never gets a break, it begins to weaken. Over time, this leads to bloating, indigestion, acid reflux, and even chronic disease. Fasting is like pressing the reset button.

Of course, fasting requires adjustment. In the beginning, you may feel hunger pangs in the morning. This is not true hunger. It is a habit. Your body has been conditioned to expect food at a certain time. Give yourself a week or two, and you will notice that those cravings fade, replaced by clarity, focus, and steady energy.

What you do during your fasting window is just as important. Hydration is key. Drink plenty of spring water, cold pressed apple juice, coffee (recommended decaf) with dairy free creamers, or herbal tea (if needed, use agave, or date syrup for natural sweeteners). These keep you refreshed without breaking your fast. Then, when your eating window begins, focus on nutrient-dense foods that nourish the body rather than burden it.

Fasting is not starvation, it is discipline. It teaches you to be in control of your appetite instead of letting your appetite control you. And in that discipline lies freedom. The truth is, when you eat is just as important as what you eat. Modern culture encourages us to snack all day and eat late into the night, but this constant feeding cycle overworks the body and robs us of health. Your digestive system needs time to rest, just like your mind and muscles. Without that rest, the gut becomes overloaded, toxins build up, and disease can begin to take root. This chapter is about reclaiming the power of timing.

***

Why You Should Stop Eating at 9 PM

Eating late at night is one of the most damaging habits for the body. Here's why:

- Digestion slows at night. Your body is preparing for rest, not heavy work. Food lingers in your stomach and ferments instead of being broken down properly.
- Insulin rises. Late eating spikes blood sugar, which is stored as fat while you sleep.
- Sleep suffers. The body wastes energy on digestion instead of deep repair.
- Toxins build. The liver, which normally detoxes during sleep, is too busy processing food.

Think of your body like a temple that closes its doors for the night. After 9 PM, let the temple rest.

***

The Power of Intermittent Fasting

The body thrives when given periods of fasting. This doesn't mean starvation, it means giving your digestive system space to reset.

Here's a simple fasting schedule:

- Stop eating by 9 PM (or earlier if possible).
- Skip breakfast.
- First meal at 12 PM (or 11 AM if you must take medication).
- Eat your last meal before 9 PM again.

This creates a 15-hour fasting window, which gives your body time to repair cells, burn stored fat instead of sugar, heal the gut and reduce inflammation.

***

What Happens When You Fast

- At 12 hours: The body begins burning fat instead of sugar.
- At 14-16 hours: Cells begin repairing themselves (autophagy).
- At 18-24 hours: Deep cleansing of the gut, toxins removed, energy levels rise.

You don't have to go extreme, just skipping breakfast and avoiding late-night snacks can change your health dramatically.

***

Food Timing and Hormones

Your hormones are tied to natural rhythms. When you eat late, you disrupt these rhythms.

- Melatonin rises at night to prepare you for sleep. Eating interferes with it.
- Insulin spikes at the wrong time, leading to diabetes risk.
- Cortisol (the stress hormone) stays high when digestion is overloaded, preventing deep rest.

Eating on time restores balance to your entire body.

Practical Tips to Stop Late Eating

1. Brush your teeth after dinner. The clean mouth signals the kitchen is closed.

2. Drink herbal tea instead. Ginger, peppermint, raspberry, chamomile, sage or hibiscus teas calm the body without calories.

3. Journal your cravings. If you want food late at night, ask yourself if it's true hunger or habit.

4. Prepare your last meal mindfully. A balanced dinner (fruit, fiber, vegetables, healthy fats) helps you stay full.

5. Go to bed earlier. The later you stay awake, the more temptation arises.

***

Resetting Your Eating Window

If you're used to eating late, it may take time to adjust. Start with small steps:

- Close the kitchen at 10 PM for one week.
- Then move it to 9:30 PM the next week.
- Finally, stick to 9 PM consistently.

The consistency will transform your digestion, your sleep, and your energy.

***

Action Steps for Chapter 2

1. Commit to no food after 9 PM starting tonight.

2. Try a 12 PM first meal for one week. Notice your energy levels.

3. Replace late night snacks with herbal tea.

4. Keep a journal to record how your body feels in the morning compared to nights when you ate late.

Chapter Three

Dead Food vs. Living Food

"If it came from a plant, eat it. If it was made in a plant, don't."
–Michael Pollan

Not all food is created equal. Some food brings life, energy, and vitality. Other food brings heaviness, sickness, and disease. The difference lies in whether the food is living or dead.

Living food is fresh, colorful, and full of nutrients. Think of fruits, vegetables, seeds, nuts, legumes, and whole grains. They are packed with vitamins, minerals, and enzymes that the body recognizes and uses with ease. When you eat living food, you feel lighter, clearer, and more energized. Dead food, on the other hand, is stripped of its life force. Processed meats, packaged snacks, sodas, white flour, white rice, white sugar, all of these have been refined, preserved, or chemically altered until very little real nutrition remains. The longer food can sit on a shelf without spoiling, the less life it contains for you.

Think about tomatoes. Fresh off the vine, it is juicy, full of color, and loaded with vitamin C and antioxidants. Now compare it to a tomato flavored chip. That chip may last months in a bag, but it contains no real tomato nutrients, just chemicals designed to mimic taste. One feeds your body, the other feeds addiction.

The food industry is not designed to keep you healthy; it's designed to keep you buying. When you walk through a grocery store, most of what you see on the shelves isn't real food at all. It's a carefully engineered product built for shelf life, flavor manipulation, and addiction. The truth is simple: if your food can sit on a shelf for years without rotting, it's not nourishing your body, it's slowly damaging it.

***

Dead Food vs. Living Food

- Food is meant to carry life. Fresh fruits, vegetables, herbs, nuts, seeds, and grains are alive with enzymes, vitamins, and minerals. But once food has been heavily processed, packaged, and pumped with preservatives, it is no longer living. It's "dead food."
- Dead food = canned goods, fast food, frozen dinners, white bread, candy, processed meats.
- Living food = raw fruits, leafy greens, sprouted grains, fresh herbs, whole veg-

etables.

Dead food fills the stomach but starves the body. Living food nourishes and heals.

***

The Protein Myth

For decades, we've been told meat is the best source of protein. But let's look closer.

- Meat is dead tissue. Once the animal is killed and the flesh is processed, the protein is denatured and stripped of much of its natural life force.
- Additives, dyes, and preservatives are mixed in to keep it looking fresh.
- Real usable protein, the kind your body needs, comes from plants, where animals get their protein in the first place.

Think about it: cows, elephants, and gorillas are all plant eaters, yet they are strong and muscular. They get protein from the earth, not from other animals. Plant protein is alive, bioavailable, and easier to digest.

***

The Danger of White Foods

Anything white and processed is a warning sign. These foods have been stripped of nutrients, bleached, or refined until they offer little more than empty calories. A powerful way to reclaim your health is to cut out white foods. Examples of harmful white foods:

- White sugar
- White flour
- White rice

- White pasta
- White bread
- White salt (refined table salt) Why they're bad:
- Cause blood sugar spikes, leading to diabetes risk.
- Feed harmful gut bacteria and yeast.
- Contribute to weight gain and inflammation.
- Offer no real nutrition, just calories.

These foods have been stripped of fiber, vitamins, and minerals. What remains are empty calories that spike blood sugar, inflame the body, and leave you craving more. Replacing these with whole grains, brown or black rice, quinoa, natural sweeteners, and fresh produce create a dramatic difference in energy and digestion. Your body is alive. It needs living fuel; not dead matter preserved with chemicals.

The choice is simple: eat food that rots quickly, because that means it still carries life. Avoid food that can sit on a shelf for years, because that means it is already dead.

Swap white foods for their natural versions:

- White sugar → agave, dates, or maple syrup (not pancake syrup).
- White flour → chickpea flour, almond flour, or coconut flour.
- White rice → quinoa, wild rice, or black or brown rice.
- White bread → sprouted or whole grain bread.
- Refined salt → pink Himalayan or sea salt.

***

Preservatives and Additives: Silent Killers

Food is supposed to spoil. That's what makes it real. If something can sit in your pantry for years, it's because chemicals are keeping it from breaking down. Those same chemicals are breaking you down. Common additives and their dangers:

- Nitrates & nitrites - linked to cancer, are found in processed meats.
- BHT/BHA - artificial preservatives linked to tumors.
- MSG - overstimulates brain cells, causes headaches and cravings.
- Artificial dyes - linked to hyperactivity, cancer, and organ stress.

The scary truth: many of these additives are also used in non-food products like plastics, fuels, or cleaning chemicals. Would you knowingly eat motor oil? Then why eat the same chemicals hidden in your snacks?

***

Learning the Real Purpose of Food

Food was never meant to be entertainment. It was meant to be medicine, fuel, and nourishment.

- Food should energize you, not make you sleepy.
- Food should heal you, not create disease.
- Food should bring clarity, not brain fog.

The truth is, the closer your food is to the earth, the closer you are to health.

***

Action Steps for Chapter 3

1. Go through your pantry and remove one dead, processed "shelf-life" food this week.

2. Replace it with a living food alternative.

3. Swap at least one white food with a whole, natural version.

4. Start reading labels, not just for the calories, but the ingredients.

5. If you can't pronounce it, ask yourself why you're eating it.

Chapter Four

The Gut - Where Health Begins

"Disease begins in the gut."

Hippocrates

Your gut is more than just a tube that digests food. It is the control center for your health. Inside your digestive tract lives trillions of tiny organisms like bacteria, fungi, and microbes that together form your gut microbiome. This community is like an ecosystem, and when it is in balance, your entire body thrives. When it is disturbed, illness follows.

The gut does far more than digest. It houses over 70% of your immune system. It communicates with your brain through the vagus nerve, influencing mood, focus, and emotions. In fact, many scientists now call the gut the "second brain." If you suffer from anxiety, depression, or constant fatigue, your gut health may be playing a bigger role than you realize.

But here's the problem: modern diets destroy gut health. Processed foods, sugar, antibiotics, artificial sweeteners, and preservatives all disrupt the delicate balance of bacteria in the gut. When harmful bacteria overgrow and beneficial bacteria die off, the lining of the gut can weaken. This condition, sometimes called "leaky gut," allows toxins and undigested particles to leak into the bloodstream, triggering inflammation, allergies, autoimmune disorders, and even chronic disease.

The good news? The gut can heal. And when it does, your entire body begins to repair. The most credible healers have all agreed: *disease begins in the gut.* Science is finally catching up to this timeless truth. When your gut is healthy, your whole body thrives. When your gut is damaged, disease begins.

***

The Gut as Your Second Brain

Did you know your gut has more nerve cells than your spinal cord? It even makes its own neurotransmitters, like serotonin, the happy hormone. This is why scientists call the gut the second brain. Your gut literally talks to your brain every single day.

A healthy gut → stable mood, strong immunity, sharp mind.

An unhealthy gut → depression, fatigue, inflammation, chronic illness.

***

How the Gut Gets Damaged

Modern eating habits are gut-destroyers. Here's what hurts your microbiome:

- Processed foods - loaded with preservatives, chemicals, and sugar.
- Antibiotics - kill not only bad bacteria, but the good bacteria too.
- Sugar & white foods - feed harmful yeast and parasites.
- Artificial sweeteners - disrupt gut bacteria balance.
- Stress - raises cortisol, which damages digestion.
- Lack of fiber - starves good bacteria.

Over time, these factors cause irritable bowel syndrome (IBS):, symptoms such as bloating, abdominal pain, and irregular bowel movements can be triggered or worsened by diet.

***

Signs of an Unhealthy Gut

- Sugar cravings
- Constant bloating or gas
- Brain fog
- Frequent sickness
- Skin issues (acne, eczema, rashes)
- Autoimmune conditions
- Fatigue, no matter how much you sleep

If you live with any of these, your gut is calling for help.

***

Healing the Gut

The good news is the gut can heal. Like a garden, it just needs the right environment.

1. **Remove the irritants**
   - Cut processed foods, white flour, sugar, and artificial additives.
   - Avoid overeating late at night.
   - Reduce alcohol and unnecessary medications when possible.

2. **Add healing foods**
   - Fermented foods: sauerkraut, kimchi, kefir, miso. leafy greens.
   - Prebiotic fibers: chickpeas, onions, asparagus, bananas, apples.
   - Herbal teas: peppermint, ginger, raspberry for soothing digestion.

- Sea moss gel heals gut lining.

3. **Restore balance**
    - Take a high-quality probiotic.
    - Eat a variety of plants daily to feed diverse gut bacteria.
    - Hydrate with spring water, coconut water, cold-pressed fruit or vegetable juices and herbal teas.
    - Hydrate with spring water, coconut water, cold-pressed fruit or vegetable juices and herbal teas.
    - Remove all dairy products from your eating habits.

4. **Reduce stress**
    - Breathe deeply before meals.
    - Exercise and stretch daily for circulation.

- Practice meditation, yoga or journaling.

***

Gut Health and Chronic Disease

Every major disease has roots in the gut.

- Diabetes – blood sugar imbalance starts with gut bacteria.
- Obesity – harmful microbes trigger overeating and fat storage.
- Autoimmune disease – leaky gut confuses the immune system.
- Depression/Anxiety – poor gut health means poor serotonin production.
- Cancer – chronic inflammation in the gut can lead to mutations.

The gut is ground zero. Heal it, and you prevent disease before it starts. Your gut is like soil. If the soil is healthy, plants grow strong. If the soil is polluted, plants wither. The same is true for you. Heal your gut, and you heal your life.

***

Action Steps for Chapter 4

1. Eliminate one gut-damaging food (soda, white bread, candy) this week.

2. Add one gut-healing food daily (like sauerkraut or garlic).

3. Drink herbal tea after dinner instead of snacking late.

4. Keep a gut journal: track bloating, energy, and mood each day.

5. Notice the connection.

Chapter Five

Exercise - Moving Your Temple

"Those who think they have no time for bodily exercise will sooner or later have to find time for illness."

Edward Stanley

The human body was built to move. Every joint, every muscle, every organ depends on motion for health. Yet in today's world, movement has been replaced by stillness. We sit in cars, sit at desks, sit on couches, and then wonder why our backs ache, our energy is low, and our minds feel clouded. The truth is simple: without movement, the body withers. With movement, the body thrives.

Exercise is not just about weight loss or appearance. It is medicine. Just 20 to 30 minutes of daily movement can transform your health. Walking after meals improves digestion and stabilizes blood sugar. Strength training builds muscle that protects your joints and burns fat naturally. Stretching relieves stress stored in the body and keeps your spine and hips flexible.

Science has shown that exercise reduces the risk of heart disease, diabetes, cancer, and depression. It strengthens the immune system and even boosts the health of your mitochondria, the tiny power plants in your cells that create energy. In other words, exercise helps you feel alive on a cellular level.

I remember talking to my landscaper, Antonio, who is 64 years old and owns a successful Landscaping Company. He complained of being too tired to exercise. His doctor insisted he walk for thirty minutes a day. At his lowest point, Antonio began daily walks in his neighborhood and within two weeks, he noticed the daily walks gave him more energy, not less. Encouraged, Antonio said he added daily stretching and light weights twice a week. Within three months, he had dropped more than 15 pounds, his blood pressure normalized, and he described feeling ten years younger. The movement and restrictions that once seemed impossible became the medicine his body craved.

Exercise doesn't need to mean gym membership or hours of sweat. It can be as simple as dancing in your living room, stretching in the morning, or doing push-ups against the wall. The key is consistency. Movement is a daily investment in your future health. You were never designed to sit still all day. Your body is a temple, and movement is the way you keep that temple strong, energized, and alive. Exercise isn't about punishment or chasing a perfect body. It's about honoring your design. Just 20 to 30 minutes a day of movement can completely transform your health, mood, and energy.

***

Why Exercise Matters

When you move, you don't just strengthen muscles, you activate life on a cellular level. Exercise:

- Improves blood circulation, delivering oxygen to every cell.
- Activates the lymphatic system, your body's natural detox system.
- Reduces stress and balances hormones.
- Strengthens the immune system.
- Keeps joints flexible and bones strong.
- Improves gut health and digestion.

Even better, exercise wakes up the mitochondria, the power plants of your cells. The more you move, the more energy your body creates. Your temple needs movement, not machines. You don't need an expensive gym membership to be healthy. Your temple thrives on simple, consistent movement like:

- Walking or light jogging
- Stretching or yoga
- Body weight exercises like squats, push-ups, pull ups or planks
- Dancing to music in your living room
- Bike riding
- Jumping rope or shadowboxing

The key is consistency, not intensity.

***

The 30-Minute Rule

If you can commit just 30 minutes a day, you'll unlock massive benefits. Here's a simple breakdown:

- 3 minutes: Warm-up (march in place, arm circles, gentle stretches).
- 25 minutes: Moderate activity (walking briskly, jogging, squats, or yoga flow).
- 2 minutes: Cool down (deep breathing, stretching, meditation).

That's it. Done daily, this routine is more powerful than hours of random exercise done inconsistently.

***

Movement as Medicine

Exercise is free medicine. It has been proven to:

- Lower blood sugar (preventing diabetes).
- Improve cholesterol and blood pressure.
- Reduce inflammation.
- Boost mood and fight depression.
- Add years to your life.

If this were a pill, it would be the most prescribed drug in the world. But unlike pills, exercise has no negative side effects, only benefits.

***

Tips for Building the Habit

1. Start small. Begin with 10 minutes a day and work up to 20–30.

2. Make it fun. Choose movement you actually enjoy.

3. Be consistent. Schedule exercise like an appointment you can't miss.

4. Listen to your body. Push gently, but don't punish yourself.

5. Mix it up. Walk one day, stretch the next, dance, ride a bike or yoga another.

***

Exercise and the Mind

Movement isn't just about the body. It also clears the mind. A short walk can calm stress, spark creativity, and reconnect you with yourself. When you treat your body as a temple, movement becomes an act of worship instead of a chore.

***

Action Steps for Chapter 5

1. Commit to 20 minutes of movement daily this week.
2. Choose one "temple practice" you enjoy (walking, stretching, biking) etc.
3. End each exercise session with 2 minutes of deep breathing.
4. Journal how your energy and mood change after each session.

Chapter Six

Reading Labels Like a Detective

If you want to break the love affair with food, you have to stop being fooled by labels. Food companies know most people glance quickly at the front of a package, skimming for words like low fat, all natural or sugar free thinking these are healthy foods. But the truth of a product is never on the front. It's in the fine print on the back. Reading labels is like detective work. Once you learn to decode ingredients, you'll see food for what it really is. Either nourishment or poison.

***

Why Labels Lie

"Low fat" usually means high sugar. "Sugar free" often hides artificial sweeteners that damage the gut. "All natural" doesn't mean healthy. It's just a marketing term. "Fortified" often means the natural nutrition was stripped away, then sprayed back in artificially. If the package has to scream how healthy it is, it usually isn't.

***

The Golden Rule: Ingredients First

The most important part of the label is not calories, not carbs, not fat grams. It's the ingredients list. Here are some rules to remember:

1. *Shorter is better.* If there are more than 10 ingredients, be cautious.

2. *Know what you're reading.* If you can't pronounce it, your body can't process it.

3. *First ingredient matters most.* Ingredients are listed by quantity–the first ones make up most of the product.

4. *Beware of sneaky sugars.* Sugar hides under names like sucrose, dextrose, corn syrup, cane juice, maltodextrin, and high fructose corn syrup.

***

Common Label Tricks

- *Different names for the same thing.* Food companies use five to six different sugars, so sugar doesn't appear first on the list.
- *Serving size manipulation.* A tiny serving makes the numbers look lower, but no one eats just that amount.
- *Healthy sounding names.* Vegetable oil

sounds good, but it's usually highly processed soybean or canola oil.

***

Ingredients Found in Non-Food Products

One of the most shocking truths is that many additives in your food are also used in industrial products. For example:

- *Propylene glycol* - used in antifreeze and in some ice creams.
- *Titanium dioxide* - used in paint, also in candies for whitening.
- *High-fructose corn syrup* - found in soda, also in cough syrup.
- *Carrageenan* - used in cosmetics, also added to dairy substitutes.

Would you put paint or antifreeze in your body? Then why eat foods laced with the same chemicals?

***

Becoming a Label Detective

When you pick up a package, ask yourself:

1. Do I recognize every ingredient?
2. Is this closer to nature or closer to a science lab?
3. Would my great-grandparents recognize this as food?

If the answer is no, put it back.

Tools for Smarter Choices

- Shop the outer aisles of the store for produce, grains, and fresh foods.

- Avoid the inner aisles where packaged products dominate.
- Use apps that scan barcodes to flag harmful ingredients.
- Practice cooking simple meals at home so you can control every ingredient.

***

Action Steps for Chapter 6

1. This week, choose three products in your pantry and write down every ingredient. Research one you don't recognize.
2. Compare the front label to the ingredient list. Pay attention to the tricks.
3. Make one swap: replace a packaged item with fresh whole food.
4. Start carrying a "label rule" in your mind: *If I can't pronounce it, I don't eat it.*

Chapter Seven

The Top 10 Dangerous Ingredients in Food

"If you can't pronounce it, you probably shouldn't eat it."

Vani Hari

The modern food industry is designed for profit, not health. Food manufacturers add chemicals to make products last longer, taste better, or look more appealing on shelves but these same ingredients can slowly destroy the body. Many of the illnesses we face today like cancer, diabetes, heart disease, and autoimmune disorders are fueled by toxic additives hidden in everyday foods.

Learning to read labels is an act of self-defense. Once you recognize the top harmful ingredients, you can avoid them and protect your health. Most of the sickness in our modern world isn't caused by fate, it's caused by what we put in our mouths every day. Food companies pack products with chemicals designed to preserve, sweeten, color, or flavor food, but they end up destroying health in the process. Here are the top ten ingredients most linked to cancer, diabetes, and chronic illness. If you do nothing else, start cutting these from your diet today.

High-Fructose Corn Syrup (HFCS)

1. Found in: sodas, candy, breads, sauces, cereals.

2. What it does: Overloads the liver, turns into fat, spikes insulin, and feeds cancer cells.

3. Why it's harmful: Unlike natural sugar, HFCS is processed so heavily that the body can't regulate it properly.

Artificial Sweeteners (Aspartame, Sucralose, Saccharin)

1. Found in: "diet" sodas, sugar-free gum, protein powders, flavored waters.

2. What it does: Confuses the body, disrupts gut bacteria, and increases cravings.

3. Why it's harmful: Linked to headaches, seizures, and cancers in animal studies.

Monosodium Glutamate (MSG)

1. Found in: chips, frozen dinners, soups, fast food.

2. What it does: Overstimulates brain cells until they burn out.

3. Why it's harmful: Causes headaches, brain fog, and addictive food cravings.

Hydrogenated Oils (Trans Fats)

1. Found in: margarine, fried foods, baked goods, packaged snacks.

2. What it does: Clogs arteries, raises bad cholesterol, lowers good cholesterol.

3. Why it's harmful: Strongly linked to heart disease, obesity, and inflammation.

Sodium Nitrates & Nitrites

1. Found in: bacon, hot dogs, deli meats, sausages.

2. What it does: Preserves meat and makes it look fresh.

3. Why it's harmful: When cooked, they form **nitrosamines**–potent cancer-causing chemicals.

Artificial Dyes (Red 40, Yellow 5, Blue 1, etc.)

1. Found in: candies, sodas, cereals, energy drinks.
2. What it does: Adds "fun" color but no nutrition.
3. Why it's harmful: Linked to hyperactivity in children, allergies, and tumors.

Potassium Bromate

1. Found in: breads, rolls, pizza dough.
2. What it does: Makes dough rise higher and whiter.
3. Why it's harmful: Classified as a possible human carcinogen; banned in many countries but still used in the U.S.

BHA & BHT (Butylated Hydroxyanisole / Hydroxytoluene)

1. Found in: chips, cereals, chewing gum, butter spreads.

2. What it does: Preserves fats and oils.

3. Why it's harmful: Linked to cancer in animal studies and endocrine disruption.

Titanium Dioxide

1. Found in: candies, gum, coffee creamers, powdered donuts.

2. What it does: Whitens and brightens food.

3. Why it's harmful: Linked to inflammation, DNA damage, and immune disruption.

Excess Refined Sugar

1. Found in: nearly everything-sauces, breads, condiments, snacks.

2. What it does: Spikes insulin, feed harmful gut bacteria, and weakens the immune system.

3. Why it's harmful: The #1 driver of obesity, diabetes, and cancer.

How to Protect Yourself

1. Read labels every time.
2. Cook more meals at home.
3. Choose whole foods: fruits, vegetables, beans, herbs, whole grains.
4. Remember: if it has a long shelf life, it's shortening **your** life.

Action Steps for Chapter 7

1. Go to your kitchen and find at least one product with one of the above ingredients. Remove it today.
2. Replace one item a week with a clean, whole-food version.
3. Start a "Never Again" list of ingredients you refuse to eat.
4. Share what you've learned with one person, saving a life begins with awareness.

Chapter Eight

Preventing & Reversing Diabetes

"A healthy body is worth more than any dollar amount."

Dr. Sebi

For many people, food is more than fuel. It becomes comfort, companionship, and even a source of emotional escape. From childhood celebrations with cake to late night snacks during loneliness, food is tied to our deepest memories and emotions. But when eating shifts from nourishment to dependency, it can feel like being trapped in a toxic love affair.

Emotional eating is one of the biggest barriers to health. We don't eat because we are hungry. We eat because we are stressed, sad, bored, or even happy. But the comfort is short lived. Afterward, guilt, bloating, or fatigue set in. The cycle repeats, and food becomes both the "lover" and the "enemy."

Ending this love affair doesn't mean rejecting food altogether. It means redefining the relationship. Food is not meant to seduce or control you. It is meant to nourish, heal, and energize you. The moment you realize that food stops being your master and becomes your servant. Here are a few truths that help break free:

- Food is not therapy. True healing comes from rest, movement, connection, and purpose, not from sugar or snacks.

- Cravings are signals, not commands. A craving for sweets may mean your body needs magnesium or hydration.

- Eating with awareness changes everything. When you slow down, chew, and taste your food, you begin to eat less but enjoy it more.

- You are in control. Food does not jump into your mouth; every bite is a choice.

Most diseases don't appear overnight. They grow silently for years, fed by daily habits, until finally symptoms can no longer be ignored. The good news is that many of these illnesses, especially diabetes, can be prevented, managed, and even reversed with the right approach.

The body has an incredible ability to heal itself if we stop damaging it and start nourishing it. When you let go of the "love affair," you create room for a new relationship where food supports your purpose instead of distracting you from it.

Diabetes: A Lifestyle Disease

Diabetes is not just about too much sugar. It's a condition where the body can no longer process sugar properly because insulin, the hormone that moves sugar from blood into cells, isn't working right. Two main causes:

1. *Insulin resistance* - cells stop responding to insulin because of constant sugar overload.
2. *Beta cell burnout* - the pancreas gets tired from producing too much insulin.

Both causes are fueled by diet, lack of movement, and processed foods.

How to Prevent or Reverse Diabetes Naturally

1. Intermittent Fasting

Skipping breakfast and eating your first meal at 12 PM (or 11 AM if needed) helps regulate blood sugar. Fasting gives the pancreas rest and lowers insulin resistance. No eating after 9 PM prevents sugar spikes.

2. *Healing Foods*

- Leafy greens - cleanse the blood and regulate sugar.
- Berries – sweet but low in sugar, packed with antioxidants.
- Beans & lentils - high fiber, stabilize blood sugar.
- Healthy fats - avocados, nuts, cooking with olive or avocado oil slow sugar absorption.
- Herbs & spices - rosemary, fenugreek, ginger all lower inflammation and support blood sugar balance.

3. *Herbal Allies*

Nature provides powerful tools for controlling blood sugar:

- Ceylon Cinnamon - improves insulin sensitivity.
- Fenugreek seeds - lower glucose levels naturally.
- Bitter melon - acts like natural insulin.
- Gymnema sylvestre - called the "sugar destroyer" in Ayurvedic medicine.
- Herbal teas - green tea, hibiscus, and dandelion support blood sugar and detox.
- Rosemary - control blood sugar

4. Movement as Medicine

- Exercise 20–30 minutes daily.
- Walking after meals lowers blood sugar spikes.

- Strength training builds muscle, which soaks up glucose from the blood.
- Movement isn't optional for diabetes. It's lifesaving!

5. *Reduce Stress*

- Stress raises cortisol, which spikes blood sugar.
- Practice meditation, deep breathing, or affirmations.
- Sleep 7–9 hours a night for hormone balance.

Other Chronic Diseases and the Gut

The same habits that prevent diabetes also protect against:

- **Heart disease** – lowered by whole foods and daily movement.

- **Cancer** - reduced inflammation and sugar intake starve cancer cells.
- **Obesity** - fasting and whole foods naturally balance weight.
- **Autoimmune disorders** - gut healing reduces flare ups.

The Power of Prevention

It's easier to prevent illness than to treat it. Your body is designed for health, not disease. Every time you eat, move, or rest, you are either moving toward health or away from it.

Action Steps for Chapter 8

1. Begin fasting stop eating at 9 PM, first meal at 12 PM (or 11 AM).
2. Add one healing food and one healing herb daily.

3. Walk for 10 minutes after at least one meal per day.

4. Drink one cup of blood sugar balancing tea (like raspberry or hibiscus) daily.

5. Write a prevention plan: list 3 small changes you'll commit to this week.

6. Pick one day a week and juice all fruit and/ or vegetables for each meal.

Chapter Nine

Herbal Medicine & Natural Healing

"Nature itself is the best physician."

Hippocrates

Long before pills and pharmacies, healing was found in plants. Across cultures and centuries, people turned to herbs, teas, and natural remedies to restore balance in the body. Today, science is rediscovering what ancient traditions already knew: nature holds powerful medicine for those who use it wisely.

Herbal teas and herbs do more than comfort. They support digestion, calm the mind, reduce inflammation, and even strengthen the immune system. Unlike processed foods or synthetic drugs, they work with the body's natural rhythms instead of against them.

Every culture around the world has used herbs, teas, and tinctures to prevent illness and restore balance. Today, many of those traditions are being rediscovered. Herbal medicine doesn't just mask symptoms. It works with the body to bring it back into harmony.

***

The Power of Plants

Plants carry compounds that support the body naturally:

- Polyphenols – fight inflammation.

- Alkaloids – energize and heal.
- Essential oils (lavender, eucalyptus or peppermint) – protect against bacteria and viruses.
- Minerals & vitamins – restore what processed food strips away.

When you drink a cup of herbal tea, you're not just hydrating. You're feeding your cells living medicine.

***

Herbal Teas for Healing

- Peppermint tea – soothes digestion and reduces bloating.
- Chamomile tea – calms the nervous system, supports sleep.
- Hibiscus tea – lowers blood pressure

and balances blood sugar.

- Ginger tea – reduces nausea, inflammation, and boosts immunity.
- Green tea – packed with antioxidants, energizes the mind.

Drinking herbal teas daily is one of the simplest ways to bring balance back to your body. Use sweeteners like agave, date syrup, maple syrup or raw honey.

***

Healing Herbs

- Ashwagandha – reduces stress and supports adrenal health.
- Holy basil (Tulsi) – supports immunity and balances blood sugar.
- Dandelion root – cleanses the liver and

supports digestion.

- Echinacea - boosts immune system, fights infections.
- Milk thistle – regenerates liver cells.
- Soursop – fights cancer, relieves anxiety and inflammation.
- Sea Moss - thyroid, heart health, skin health.
- Chlorophyll - boosts red blood cells, supports digestion.
- Muira Puama - often called potency wood, balances mood & boosts libido naturally.
- Maca – supports hormonal balance and reproductive health in men & women.
- Dong Quai - balance hormones, treats menopause and menstrual cycle.

These herbs can be used in teas, capsules, gel or tinctures depending on preference.

Tinctures: Concentrated Healing

Tinctures are liquid extracts of herbs, usually made with alcohol or glycerin. Because they are concentrated, they act quickly in the body. Just a few drops under the tongue can deliver powerful plant medicine.

- Echinacea tincture - boosts immune defense.
- Valerian root tincture - promotes deep sleep.
- Ginkgo Biloba tincture - improves blood flow to the brain.
- Ginseng tincture - increases energy and focus.
- Gota Kola tincture - improves blood

flow to the brain, memory and concentration.

Marijuana as Medicine

Long before it was used recreationally, cannabis was medicine. Its compounds, **THC** and **CBD,** interact with the body's endocannabinoid system, which helps regulate pain, mood, and inflammation.

- CBD (non-psychoactive): reduces anxiety, inflammation, seizures, and chronic pain.
- THC: useful for nausea, appetite stimulation, and pain relief.

Caution: Not all strains are the same, and quality matters. Modern strains are often hybrids, so effects can vary. Always seek natural, clean sources, not chemically altered products.

Building a Natural Wellness Cabinet

Instead of filling your shelves with pills and chemicals, build a wellness cabinet of herbs and teas:

- Peppermint, ginger, and raspberry teas.
- Basil, Marjoram and Bay leaf.
- Herbal tinctures for stress, sleep, and immunity.
- Cannabis or CBD oil (where legal).
- Dried herbs for cooking and healing.

Having nature's medicine within reach before illness takes hold is the key to prevention.

***

Action Steps for Chapter 9

1. Replace one daily beverage with an herbal tea.

2. Add at least one healing herb to your meals this week.

3. Explore tinctures: try one for sleep, stress, or immunity.

4. Research marijuana/CBD laws in your area if you want to explore plant-based pain management.

5. Begin building a natural wellness cabinet at home.

Chapter Ten

The Power of Mitochondria

Your body is made up of trillions of cells. Inside each one is a tiny engine called the mitochondrion (plural: mitochondria). These engines are responsible for creating energy. In fact, every heartbeat, every breath, every movement, every thought you have is powered by your mitochondria. When your mitochondria are strong, you feel vibrant, clear headed, and energized. When they are weak or damaged, fatigue, brain fog, and disease take over. Scientists now believe mitochondrial dysfunction plays a role in diabetes,

Alzheimer's, cancer, and even premature aging. The good news? You can strengthen and protect your mitochondria with the choices you make every day.

What Are Mitochondria?

Mitochondria are often called the "powerhouses of the cell." Their job is to take the food you eat and the oxygen you breathe and turn them into ATP (adenosine triphosphate), the energy currency of the body. Without ATP, your body shuts down. Without strong mitochondria, disease takes over. Research shows that mitochondrial dysfunction is at the root of nearly every chronic illness:

- Diabetes
- Heart disease
- Cancer
- Alzheimer's

- Autoimmune disorders

If the cell's power source is weak, the entire body suffers.

***

How to Strengthen Your Mitochondria

1. Fasting

When you fast (stop eating after 9 PM and delay your first meal until 11 or 12), your body goes into repair mode. Old, weak mitochondria are broken down and replaced with new, stronger ones.

2. Exercise

Moving your body stimulates mitochondrial growth. Even 20–30 minutes a day of walking, strength training, or cycling makes a difference. While cardio increases oxygen delivery, strength training builds more mitochondria in muscle cells.

3. Eating Clean, Living Foods

Dead foods (processed, shelf stable, filled with chemicals) weaken mitochondria. Living foods such as fresh fruits, vegetables, herbs, seeds, and healthy fats, feed your cells with energy.

4. Reduce Toxins

Artificial sweeteners, preservatives, and chemical additives poison your mitochondria. So do smoking, alcohol, and environmental toxins. Reading labels and choosing clean foods directly protects your cellular engines.

5. Rest and Stress Reduction

Your mitochondria repair while you sleep. Chronic stress, poor sleep, and overwork burn them out. Meditation, deep breathing, and proper rest keep them strong.

6. Herbal and Natural Support

Certain herbs and nutrients directly support mitochondrial function:

- CoQ10 - protects and energizes mitochondria.
- Hawthorne Berry - health and blood pressure regulator.
- Green tea extract - boosts mitochondrial efficiency.
- Magnesium - vital for ATP production.
- Propolis - antioxidant, improves mitochondrial respiratory capacity.
- Mullein -respiratory and viral health.

***

Your Body: A Temple at the Cellular Level

When you say, "my body is a temple," it's the absolute truth. Every cell is a brick, and every mitochondrion is a spark of divine energy. Protect them, and your temple stands strong. Neglect them, and the foundation begins to crumble.

Action Steps for Chapter 10

1. Begin practicing overnight fasting daily.
2. Exercise at least 30 minutes a day to stimulate new mitochondria.
3. Add one mitochondria-supporting food or herb to your meals (ginger, green tea, berries).
4. Commit to 6–8 hours of sleep each night.
5. Reduce at least one toxin from your diet or environment this week.

Chapter Eleven

The Food & Meal Prep Guide

"The best preparation for tomorrow is doing your best today."

H. Jackson Brown Jr.

One of the greatest obstacles to eating healthily is not intention. It's convenient. When hunger strikes and no healthy food is ready, we reach for what is quick: fast food, processed snacks, or sugary drinks. But when your kitchen is stocked with nourishing foods and your meals are planned ahead, success becomes natural.

Meal prep is not about rigid dieting. It's about freedom. It frees you from last-minute decisions, stress, and unhealthy compromises. Think of it as creating a supportive environment where your future self always wins.

Knowledge is power, but action is transformation. By now, you understand the dangers of processed foods, the power of fasting, the role of herbs, and the importance of exercise. But the question remains: What should you actually eat each day?

This chapter offers a simple, realistic roadmap you can follow.

***

The Principles of Eating Well

1. Whole foods over processed foods. If it comes in a box and has a long shelf life, it's not real food.

2. Color matters. Bright fruits and vegetables mean living nutrients.

3. Balance your plate. Aim for fiber, healthy fats, plant proteins, & herbs in every meal.

4. Hydrate. Water and herbal teas should be your main beverages.

5. Listen to your body. No one diet fits all. Pay attention to how food makes you feel.

***

Sample Daily Eating Window (Intermittent Fasting)

- 9 PM – 11/12 PM: No food. Hydrate with water, fruit or vegetable juice, or herbal teas.
- 12 PM (First Meal): A clean, balanced plate.
- 3–4 PM (Snack if needed): Light and nutrient-dense.
- 6–7 PM (Dinner): Filling but not heavy.
- After 9 PM: No eating. Let your gut rest and repair.

Sample Meals Lunch Ideas

- Warm steel cut oatmeal with berries and chia seeds. (Can use quinoa as an oat replacement).
- Peanut butter smoothie with strawberries, blueberries, banana, peanut butter, date syrup, and milk (coconut, hemp oat or almond)
- Avocado or Hummus toast on whole-grain bread,
- Quinoa salad with romaine lettuce, sprouts, tomatoes, hummus, chickpeas, cucumbers, , onions, mushrooms and tahini dressing
- Bowl with black or brown rice, sauteed mushrooms, peppers, and onions, avocado, red or sweet potato and Teriyaki sauce.
- Lentil soup with curry.
- Large mixed salad with tahini or ginger dressing or any dairy free dressing.
- Wrap with barbecue Jack fruit, romaine or kale lettuce, pickled onions, tomatoes, pickles, and guacamole.

Snack Ideas

- Apple slices with almond butter
- Herbal tea with fruit and a handful of healthy nuts.(walnuts, almonds, cashews or pistachios).
- Guacamole and vegan style chips
- Fresh berries, smoothies or fresh juice.
- Raw vegetables and cashew cheese dip.

***

Dinner Ideas

- Spaghetti squash, and mixed vegetables with spaghetti or lemon herb sauce.
- Stir-fried mixed vegetables with sesame oil
- Roasted butternut squash with Brussels sprouts
- Quinoa or brown or black rice with sauteed greens and herbs

■ Butternut squash soup

***

Evening Wind-Down

■ Warm ginger or hibiscus tea to support digestion and relaxation.

Meal Prep Tips

1. Batch cook grains and beans. Make a pot of wild, black or brown rice, or quinoa, and lentils at the start of the week.

2. Chop vegetables in advance. Keep containers of ready-to-cook veggies.

3. Make spice blends. Combine oregano, marjoram, basil, rosemary, thyme, sea or pink salt, garlic, onion and parsley to flavor meals.

4. Prep teas. Brew large jars of herbal tea and keep them in the fridge.

5. Pack snacks. Nuts, seeds, fruit and vegetables prevent bad choices when having hunger strikes.

There are also meal prep service companies with healthy food options that can be ordered and delivered to your doorstep.

Herbal Teas to Rotate Weekly

- Ginger tea – digestion and inflammation.
- Peppermint tea – gut health and bloating.
- Hibiscus tea – blood sugar and pressure balance.
- Chamomile tea – stress and sleep.
- Green tea – boosts metabolism and energy.
- Raspberry tea – digestion and immune support.
- Lemongrass tea – reduces stress and anxiety.
- Sage tea – boost memory and heart health.

Foods to Avoid

- Anything white (white bread, white flour, white rice, white sugar).
- Packaged snacks with more than 5 ingredients.
- Sodas and "diet" drinks.
- Meats filled with preservatives or additives.
- Anything with words you can't pronounce on the label.

***

Action Steps for Chapter 11

1. Plan your meals for the next 3 days using the sample guide above.
2. Prep at least one batch meals this week (like lentils, rice, or chopped veggies).
3. Choose one herbal tea and drink it daily for 7 days.

4. Remove at least one "white food" from your kitchen this week.

5. Keep a food journal to track how your body responds to these changes.

Chapter Twelve

The Ingredient Dictionary

Most people don't realize that the foods on grocery store shelves are filled with substances you would never add to a home-cooked meal. Food manufacturers hide behind long, scientific names, making it hard for the average person to know what they're eating. This dictionary is your tool to fight back. Learn to read labels, pronounce the ingredients, and understand what they really do to your food, to your body, and even to non-food products.

***

How to Use This Guide

- Pronunciation: helps you sound out tricky chemical names.
- Definition: explains what the ingredient actually is.
- Body Effects: what it does to your health.
- Other Uses: where else this chemical is found (often shocking).

***

Common Food Ingredients to Watch Out For

1. **Monosodium Glutamate** (MSG)

   - Pronunciation: MON-oh-SOE-dee-um GLOO-ta-mate

- Definition: A flavor enhancer added to soups, chips, frozen meals, and sauces.
- Body Effects: Overstimulates brain cells, may cause headaches, cravings, & brain fog.
- Other Uses: Found in beauty products and even some fertilizers.

2. **High-Fructose Corn Syrup** (HFCS)

- Pronunciation: HI fruk-TOHS corn SUR-up
- Definition: A cheap, processed sweetener made from corn.
- Body Effects: Spikes insulin, overloads the liver, linked to obesity and diabetes.
- Other Uses: Used in cough syrup, processed breads, and sauces.

3. **Natural Flavors**

- Pronunciation:NAT-yur-uhl FLAY-vurz
- Definition: Mixtures from plant or animal sources used to improve or restore taste in processed foods.
- Body Effects: Highly processed; may contain solvents or preservatives. Can cause sensitivity or allergic reactions in some people.
- Other Uses: Common in perfumes, cosmetics, and supplements for added scent or flavor.

4. **Titanium Dioxide**

- Pronunciation:ty-TAY-nee-um dye-OX-ide
- Definition: A whitening agent used

in candy, powdered donuts, and coffee creamers.

- Body Effects: Linked to inflammation, DNA damage, and gut imbalance.
- Other Uses: Used in sunscreen, paint, and cosmetics.

5. **BHA** (Butylated Hydroxyanisole) & BHT (Butylated Hydroxytoluene)

- Pronunciation:BYOO-ti-lay-ted hi-DROX-ee-ANN-iss-ole / hi-DROX-ee-TOE-loo-een
- Definition: Preservatives added to oils, cereals, chips, and chewing gum.
- Body Effects: Hormone disruptors; linked to cancer in animal studies.
- Other Uses: Used in rubber, plastics, and cosmetics.

6. **Aspartame**

- Pronunciation: *AS-par-tame*
- Definition: A widely used artificial sweetener found in diet sodas and sugar-free products.
- Body Effects: Linked to headaches, seizures, depression, and cancer in some studies.
- Other Uses: Found in pharmaceuticals like chewable vitamins and laxatives.

7. **Potassium Bromate**

- Pronunciation:POE-TASS-ee-um BRO-mate
- Definition: A chemical used to make bread rise higher and look whiter.

- Body Effects: Classified as a possible human carcinogen; banned in Europe, Japan, and Canada, but still legal in the U.S.
- Other Uses: Industrial uses in hair products and flame retardants.

8. **Carrageenan**

- Pronunciation: *CARE-ah-gee-nan*
- Definition: A thickening agent made from red seaweed, found in non-dairy milks and ice cream.
- Body Effects: Can trigger gut inflammation and digestive issues.
- Other Uses: Used in cosmetics, toothpaste, and air fresheners.

9. **Artificial Food Dyes** (Red 40, Yellow 5, Blue 1)

- Pronunciation: common color names
- Definition: Synthetic colors made from petroleum.
- Body Effects: Linked to hyperactivity in children, allergies, and cancer in lab studies.
- Other Uses: Used in cosmetics, soaps, and even industrial products.

10. **Propylene Glycol**

- Pronunciation:PROH-peh-leen GLY-call
- Definition: A thickening agent used in ice cream, salad dressings, and flavorings.

- Body Effects: Can irritate the skin, lungs, and digestive system.
- Other Uses: Main ingredient in antifreeze, e-cigarettes, and brake fluid.

The Golden Rule

If you can't pronounce it or don't know what it is, don't eat it. The body was not designed to process synthetic chemicals. The closer you stay to natural, whole foods, the stronger and healthier your body will be.

***

Action Steps for Chapter 12

1. Pick 3 ingredients from this list and check your kitchen for them. Remove at least one today.

2. Start keeping a "Do Not Eat" ingredient list on your phone for quick reference when shopping.

3. Practice reading labels every time you buy a packaged product.

4. Share this dictionary with your family. Awareness saves lives!

Chapter Thirteen

Your Body Is a Temple

Your body is more than flesh and bone. It is sacred. Just as a church or temple is treated with reverence, care, and respect, so too should your body be honored. When you mistreat your body with poor food, lack of movement, or neglect, it is as though you are allowing weeds to overgrow a sacred garden.

Many of us take better care of our cars, clothes, or houses than we do our own bodies. But unlike possessions, your body cannot be replaced. You only get one. If you wouldn't pour sugar into your car's gas tank, why pour it into your body's engine? If you wouldn't let trash pile up in your living room, why let toxins pile up in your cells?

Honoring your body as a temple means approaching health as an act of respect; for yourself, for life, and for the energy that flows through you. It is not about vanity. It is about gratitude. Every step you take, every breath you draw, is a gift. And when you care for your body, you extend the life of that gift. Your body is not an accident. It is not disposable. It is a sacred temple built to house your spirit, your energy, and your purpose.

Just like a church or place of worship, your body deserves respect, care, and reverence. Every bite of food, every breath, every movement is an offering. The way you treat your body reflects the way you treat your life. Imagine walking into a church, mosque, or temple. The floors are clean, the windows polished, the air peaceful. People lower their voices out of respect. The space itself commands care. Now imagine the opposite. A neglected building with broken glass, trash, and no light. Would you want to worship there? That's what happens when we neglect our bodies. We turn our sacred space into a dumping ground for processed foods, chemicals, stress, and disease.

Treating your body like a temple means:

1. Nourishment instead of abuse. Whole foods not processed ones.
2. Movement instead of stagnation. Exercise, stretching, and daily activity.
3. Rest instead of burnout. Sleep and silence for repair.
4. Awareness instead of ignorance. Reading labels and listening to your body.
5. Connection instead of isolation. Sharing meals, walking, or joining social groups.

When you eat clean, whole foods, you honor the Creator's design. Fresh fruits, vegetables, herbs, juicing, and teas are gifts of the earth. They are medicine and life. When you eat processed, chemical filled products, you dishonor your body and shorten your life. Food can be an act of worship or an act of destruction. The choice is yours.

***

The Spiritual Side of Health

Health is not just physical. It is mental, emotional, and spiritual. Fasting strengthens discipline. Exercise clears the mind. Herbal teas calm the spirit. Respect for your body deepens respect for your life. When you care for your temple, you connect more deeply with God, with nature, and with yourself.

***

The Final Choice

This book has given you tools: fasting, mindful eating, exercise, herbs, meal prep, ingredient awareness, and healing practices. But none of it matters unless you make a choice. Ask yourself today: Will I continue treating my body like a trash can or will I honor it as a temple? The answer will determine not just your health, but your future.

Action Steps for Chapter 13

1. Write down one way you've been dishonoring your body. Commit to changing it this week.

2. Choose one daily ritual that honors your body as a temple (morning tea, prayer walk, meditation).

3. Visit a quiet place of worship (or create one in your home) and reflect on how you can bring that same respect to your body.

4. Share your health journey with someone else. Inspiration multiplies when it's passed on.

Your body is the only place you will ever live. Guard it, feed it, move it, and honor it. In doing so, you protect your energy, your spirit, and your purpose.

Chapter Fourteen

Sample 7-Day Meal Plan

Mindful Meals to Reset, Refuel, and Reconnect with Your Body

Each day in this plan focuses on nourishment–whole-food ingredients, balanced energy, and mindful eating. Portions are flexible; eat until you are satisfied, not full. Drink plenty of water and herbal teas throughout the day.

Day 1

Lunch: Quinoa Salad with Kale and Chick-peas

Instructions: Cook quinoa, chop kale or romaine, cook chickpeas, cherry tomatoes, cucumber, olive oil, lemon juice, sea salt, and pepper.. Toss all ingredients together in a large bowl. Massage the kale until tender, drizzle with olive oil and lemon juice, and season to taste.

Snack (3 PM): Apple with Almond Butter. Slice a crisp apple and serve with one to two tablespoons of natural almond butter. Eat slowly to enjoy the texture and sweetness.

Dinner: Jack fruit bowl with Quinoa

Instructions: Add water to a medium saucepan, boil jack fruit for 10 minutes (squeeze lemon or lime into water. Cook quinoa, Sauté mushrooms, peppers and onions (optional). Sauté jack fruit with your choice of seasoning. Combine all ingredients into a bowl, Add diced tomatoes and cucumbers, crispy fried onions strings, coleslaw (dairy free) and sweet barbecue sauce.

Day 2

Lunch: Black or Brown Rice Bowl with Black Beans and Avocado

Instructions: Combine warm brown rice with black beans, sliced avocado, sweet peas, and a spoonful of salsa. Garnish with lime juice and fresh cilantro.

Snack: Walnuts and Hibiscus Tea. Enjoy a small handful of walnuts with a cup of hibiscus tea for antioxidants and heart-supportive fats.

Dinner: Ginger Sesame Stir Fried Vegetables

Instructions: Sauté mixed vegetables such as bell peppers, onions, carrots broccoli, and snap peas in sesame oil with fresh ginger and a splash of low-sodium soy sauce or tamari.

Day 3

Lunch: Chickpea Curry with Spinach and Coconut Milk

Instructions: Sauté onion and garlic, then add chickpeas, curry powder, and coconut milk. Stir in spinach until wilted. Serve warm over brown rice or quinoa.

Snack: Fresh Berries. A cup of strawberries, blueberries, or raspberries makes a light and refreshing antioxidant-rich snack.

Dinner: Roasted Sweet Potatoes with Steamed Green Beans

Instructions: Roast cubed sweet potatoes at 400°F with olive oil and sea salt. Steam green beans and toss with a small amount of garlic and pepper.

Day 4

Lunch: Kale and Bell Pepper Salad with Tahini Dressing

Instructions: Combine chopped kale, bell peppers, cucumbers, and hemp seeds. Whisk tahini, lemon juice, water, garlic, and salt for the dressing. Drizzle over the salad and toss until evenly coated.

Snack: Pumpkin Seeds and Green Tea

Enjoy one-fourth cup of pumpkin seeds with a warm cup of green tea for an energizing, mineral-rich snack.

Dinner: Vegetable Stir Fry with Garlic Sauce

Instructions: Cook brown rice. Stir fry your favorite vegetables such as zucchini, mushrooms, and peppers in olive oil with minced garlic and tamari. Serve over rice.

Day 5

Lunch: Lentil and Vegetable Stew with Turmeric and Cumin

Instructions: Simmer lentils, carrots, celery, and tomatoes in vegetable broth with turmeric, cumin, and garlic until thick and fragrant.

Snack: Orange and Chamomile Tea. Peel and enjoy a fresh orange. Sip warm chamomile tea for calm focus and digestive support.

Dinner: Quinoa with Roasted Carrots and Sauteed Spinach

Instructions: Roast carrots until tender and slightly caramelized. Serve over cooked quinoa with a side of lightly sauteed spinach in olive oil and garlic.

Day 6

Lunch: Chickpea and Cucumber Salad with Olive Oil and Parsley

Instructions: Mix chickpeas, diced cucumber, fresh parsley, olive oil, and a squeeze of lemon. Add a pinch of salt and pepper to taste.

Snack: Almonds and Hibiscus Tea. Enjoy a small handful of almonds with a cup of hibiscus tea to balance blood sugar and support hydration.

Dinner: Cauliflower and Broccoli Soup with Whole Grain Garlic Bread

Instructions: Blend cooked cauliflower and broccoli with vegetable broth, garlic, and a touch of olive oil. Serve warm with toasted whole-grain bread rubbed with garlic.

Day 7

Lunch: Brown Rice and Black Bean Bowl with Avocado and Salsa

Instructions: Layer brown rice, black beans, diced avocado, fresh salsa, and cilantro. Squeeze lime on top and serve warm or chilled.

Snack: Berries and Green Tea. A small bowl of mixed berries with a cup of green tea makes a light, energizing snack.

Dinner: Roasted Sweet Potatoes, Lentils, and Spinach Salad

Instructions: Toss roasted sweet potato cubes with cooked lentils and fresh spinach. Drizzle with olive oil and lemon juice for a simple, heart-healthy meal.

This seven-day plan is not a diet; it is a reset. It teaches your body to crave nourishment over numbness, presence over distraction, and peace over punishment. Each meal is an opportunity to practice self-respect and awareness through food.

Chapter Fifteen

Appendix - Your Health Toolkit

Here is an extended ingredient dictionary with more common additives and chemicals to recognize and avoid.

1. Maltodextrin
   - Pronunciation: MAL-toh-DEX-trin
   - Definition: A processed carbohydrate used as a thickener or filler.
   - Body Effects: Spikes blood sugar like pure sugar; damages gut bacteria.
   - Other Uses: Found in supplements, in-

fant formulas, and even pesticides.

2. Guar Gum
    - Pronunciation: *GWAR gum*
    - Definition: A thickener from guar beans, found in sauces and dairy substitutes.
    - Body Effects: May cause bloating and digestive upset in sensitive people.
    - Other Uses: Used in cosmetics and industrial paper products.

3. Xanthan Gum
    - Pronunciation: *ZAN-than gum*
    - Definition: A thickener from fermented sugar, added to gluten-free products.
    - Body Effects: Can trigger gut irritation for some.

- Other Uses: Found in toothpaste, lotions, and shampoo.

4. Polysorbate 80
   - Pronunciation: POL-ee-SOR-bate 80
   - Definition: An emulsifier in ice cream, dressings, and sauces.
   - Body Effects: Disrupts gut lining, may increase risk of inflammation.
   - Other Uses: Found in vaccines, cosmetics, and cleaning products.

5. Sodium Benzoate
   - Pronunciation: SO-dee-um BEN-zo-ate
   - Definition: A preservative in sodas and condiments.
   - Body Effects: Forms benzene (a carcinogen) when combined with vitamin

C.

- Other Uses: Found in cosmetics and medicines.

***

Quick Reference–Top Rules to Live By

- Stop eating at 9 PM.
- Skip breakfast: first meal at 12 PM (11 AM if needed).
- Avoid white foods (bread, flour, sugar, rice).
- Exercise at least 20 – 30 minutes daily.
- Read every ingredient label.
- Remove toxic ingredients (MSG, nitrates, dyes, HFCS).
- Drink herbal teas daily, and juice fruit

and vegetables.

- Listen to your body, not your cravings.
- Treat your body as a temple.
- Remember: All diseases start in the gut. Heal the gut, and you heal the body.

***

Action Steps for the Appendix

1. Print out the "Top Rules to Live By" and place it on your fridge.
2. Choose one new herb or tea each week to add to your routine.
3. Use the 7-day meal plan as a starter guide, then mix and match your own.
4. Keep updating your "Do Not Eat" list as you learn more ingredients.

Chapter Sixteen

Conclusion

As you come to the end of this book, I hope you see that this journey has never been just about food, it has always been about you. About learning to listen, to heal, and to live with intention.

Breaking the love affair with food isn't about rejecting it; it's about redefining it. It's about creating a relationship built on awareness instead of impulse, and nourishment instead of emotional escape. It's realizing that what we crave most isn't always found on a plate; sometimes, it's peace, connection, or self-acceptance.

Healing is not a straight path. There will be moments of progress and moments of doubt. But every time you choose mindfulness over reaction, compassion over judgment, and purpose over habit; you reclaim a part of yourself. I started my journey towards living a plant-based lifestyle 20 years ago and it was not an easy process to give up some of the foods I thought I could not live without, but the journey and rewards have been life changing. Imagine living a lifestyle without prescription pills, aches and pains, doctor's visits and receiving a clean bill of health. This is not a judgment; it's a call to action.

My hope is these words stay with you long after you've closed this book. That you continue to ask yourself, *How important is living to me?* and that your answer inspires action, love, and growth.

Remember: You are not broken. You are becoming. And with each step toward balance, you are already living your breakthrough.

With peace and gratitude,

Amir Carter

Chapter Seventeen

Notes

www.ingramcontent.com/pod-product-compliance
Lightning Source LLC
LaVergne TN
LVHW022225200926
848481LV00006B/2122